#GONE *Girl*

31 Day Mask-Up Devotional

A Devotional Collaboration Written by Amazing Women

#GONE *Girl*

31 Day Mask-Up Devotional

A Devotional Collaboration Written by Amazing Women

EJF PUBLISHING HOUSE

CHICAGO, ILLINOIS

Angela Johnson/EJF Publishing House

#GoneGirl 31 Day Mask Up Devotional. -- 1st ed.
ISBN 978-1-7368985-2-9

TABLE OF CONTENTS

EJF PUBLISHING HOUSE

CHICAGO, ILLINOIS

FOREWORD

#Gonegirl 31 Day Mask-Up Devotional is a powerful anthology of testimonies by women of faith from all walks of life. Compiled by Pastor Angela Johnson, this book shares the experiences of women who have lost much; but, oh, through their stories we see how God has given them GREAT VICTORY!

These authors have given us a glimpse into their secret hurts and shown how God transformed their lives. From them we learn that it is not about masking your pain, masking your hurts, or masking your insecurities. It is about protecting your future, your purpose, and your destiny!

These authors are ready for their next level! They challenge every reader to start masking up to protect your gift, anointing, talent, purpose, and future by un-masking every lie of the enemy. It is time to become the woman that God has preordained you to be!

As I have read through this anthology, I have cried and smiled. I highly recommend this book. You will be encouraged and inspired as you open your heart to the amazing stories of these authors.

Desiree Fleming

Visionary Author of #GONE GIRL 31-Day Mask Up Devotional
2X Author|Radio Personality|Pastor

Although gifted and called, **Pastor Angela Johnson** did not seek to be "fully" used by God when she was a teenager. However, she persevered! It was during this time that Lorean Mccullouch (God Mom) encouraged, mentored, and made her sing and direct the choir. Eventually, her God mother asked the church to send her to music school.

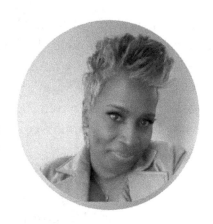

Among other key influences in her life were Pastor Carolyn Vessel, Dr. Tracey Brim, Apostles John & Rosemary Abercrombie, Evangelist Karla Greer of Co-Laborers with Christ Outreach Ministries. It was during her involvement with the ministry there that Angela not only began to manifest her gift as a psalmist, but how to "fully" believe in herself and in God.

In 1990, she began serving in ministry where her gifts were nurtured. An effective witness, Angela continued her passion of ministry through song, evangelism, and the prophetic word as minister and praise and worship leader at Truth and Deliverance Church, under the leadership of Pastors John and Rosemary Abercrombie. God later directed her to Living Word Christian Center, where she began ministering in jails and prisons throughout Illinois. In addition, Angela has assisted numerous "grass root" ministries reach the lost with the gospel.

Angela is a licensed Evangelist, ordained Pastor and Co-Founder of Greater Love, Greater Works Outreach International. She is also the Podcast Host of **OneSister2Another** heard on IHeart Radio and #Gonegirl All Women Empowerment Group-Executive Director. Her ministry was birthed out of a passion and a need to reach the unsaved and the saved with encouragement and instruction in righteousness.

She seeks to assure that in times of trouble Jesus will hide you. Most importantly her ministry is called of God to be a pillar of strength, restoring integrity and trust back into the pulpit. In addition, she is a pioneer and community leader who believes that men and women deserve a fresh start after any challenge. Pastor Angela is also a go to vessel that assist and guide ex-offenders with their reentry into society. She has been tremendously blessed with a network of friends who provide job training, education, housing, and spiritual guidance.

For the past 34 years, Angela has been employed with American Airlines, where she serves on the management team. She is also an Advisor of the "American Airline African American Employee Resource Group." Her position affords her an opportunity to take the gospel of Jesus Christ throughout the world. Angela often says, "If I can impact just **one**, that's a nation". Whether she's on the job, flying around the world, ministering in churches, or at home with her family, she's always presented with the opportunity to impact **one**.

Contact Information
Email onesister2another@gmail.com
Facebook https://www.facebook.com/profile.php?id=575511882

CHAPTER ONE

SAY YOU CAN, SAY YOU CAN'T; EITHER WAY YOU'RE RIGHT

BY PASTOR ANGELA JOHNSON

God's Word Is Powerful and Mighty. God's Word Is
Powerful and Effective. Hebrews 4:12, NLT

The enemy is always interested in making sure that as God's creation you never walk in wholeness or healing. He understands the power of words even when we don't.

Recently, I turned 56 years old and I am so grateful because I have accomplished a lot in my life. As a media host and pastor alongside the world's most amazing leader, Robert L Johnson Jr. of Greater Love, Greater Works Outreach International, I am also a contributing author to **Unleashed and Unafraid, Volume 3, Ponytail Prayers.**

Sometimes I find it strange and sometimes even terrifying when I consider all my successes. I can still remember turning 50 and being excited because I had made it to half a century. I remember witnessing my other sister-girls' journeys on this path and it always seemed they were transitioning well to their new age. As a matter of fact, I remembered thinking Well *God, what now?* The excitement I had dreamed this new age would bring me soon brought on fearful thoughts. I had thought the 50 & Fabulous party would be the proof that I had finally come into my own and established myself. The more I thought about it, the more concerned I became about my mortality. How long would I live? Would I get sick and immediately check out? All these concerns came to a head in 2019 and 2020 with the onset of the pandemic. The world was in chaos and I began to wonder if I would get Covid and die.

As it turned out, I did get Covid and lived through it. My husband, on the other hand, was hit hard. Here is where God showed me how my words carry weight on earth and in the heavens. My husband battled pneumonia and came through it. Next pancreatic challenges, like a tsunami, hit him and he came through it. He even had emergency brain surgery and came through it.

I believe today and more than ever that God had to show me why I was and who I really had become in Him. The short version is this y'all. I walked into that hospital when my husband checked in with pneumonia and said, "If he doesn't need a ventilator, he is going home with me." Although I still had Covid-19, I took him home and we nursed each other back to health.

Then came brain surgery. On my way home after officiating a service, I learned that the doctors at immediate care discovered blood in places it shouldn't have been in my husband's brain. Overwhelmed, I felt like a ton of bricks had hit me because I had just dealt with his pneumonia and pancreas attack.

As I hurried to the hospital, I remember praying, God, *please slow my racing heart.* He did and I was able to think rationally. In the back of my mind I was thinking, *Is this what 56 is going to be like, challenge after challenge?* I prayed, "God, I live for you. My husband, Pastor Robert lives for you. What is it, God?"

He spoke to me and asked, what are you saying, daughter? Immediately, the scripture that says I'm redeemed from the curses of the law came to mind. Let the redeemed of the Lord "Say So." I said, Say what?

Down in my soul, I heard God tell me to say what you want to happen next while you're still in your now! Y'all, I prayed right there for the Neurologist/Anesthesiologist. Oh yes, I did. I told them, "God's with you. You have sensitive cargo (my hubby). I need you to get it right in there." As they rolled Rob into surgery, he showed me the peace sign.

I'm in tears writing this as I remember that day. By the time my son parked his car, the doctor was calling. I picked up not really knowing what to think. I heard this voice say, "Mrs. Johnson, we're finished."

I was like, "No you're not! You have the wrong person. Read the tag on his wrist."

The doctor raised his voice. "Mrs. Johnson, your prayers worked!"

I dropped the phone. I praised God. "God I will forever live my life decreeing your loyalty to your children. Your word works even when we don't. My God!"

According to my husband, the doctors claimed there was no way he could have been this way for 8 days. They said it was important to seal the vessel in his head, but to have no irreversible damage was a miracle. I knew that my husband was truly blessed with a miracle. In fact, he was a miracle because he was born with this pocket inside his skull where all the blood that should have been creating brain damage, aneurysm, etc. had collected.

God gets all the glory! I started thinking and this is my truth. I have always felt called by God. I remember the devout Baptist church I grew up in where women were never invited into the pulpit for anything but to bring water to the minister. Today I recognize that my calling is from God and not man. Whereas I had cringed at the thought of aging and I had cringed at being this voice, I realize today after all these life's altering events that this is my time to speak up. I must speak up and maintain the position God has called me to. My calling is from God and not from man.

Whether I am 50, 60, or 70, totally culturally sharp or even poor, I am on my way to believing that I am rich on all levels. I'm convinced that according to Luke 10:19 NIV that I have power to say what the Word says with a conviction that convinces the masses.

If you say it and it lines up with the will of God, the ways of God, and His Word, may it be unto you according to your faith.

Now what? I asked, "What, God?" This is what He says loud and clear folks, "Say you can, say you can't; either way you're right!

In 2009, while living in Milwaukee, Wisconsin, with her husband and children, **Bobbie Wallace** struggled with alcohol. During that period over 10 years ago, Bobbie was arrested while she was in crisis. Fortunately, her case was adjudicated, but that was a very dark period in her family's life. She is happy to report that today both she and her husband are clean and sober. They have made Christ their personal Lord and Savior and 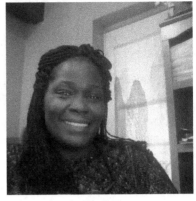 actively involved in her church City of Praise and at the Above and Beyond Family recovery center.

As often as possible, Bobbie and her husband share their story with individuals who can benefit from their journey. Bobbie was offered gainful employment with Above and Beyond and serves as their Women in Sobriety group facilitator. Additionally, she is responsible for collecting and processing patient drug screens and, more recently, took on the role of screening and processing patients for COVID-19.

Bobbie is a full-time, state-certified phlebotomist for Above and Beyond. With their assistance and support, she was accepted into the Medex EMT training program. She successfully completed her course of study as class valedictorian in December of 2020 and passed the EMT National Registration Certification. Moreover, she was offered a position with Medex as an EMT. She is maintaining this role while attending Midwestern Career College to obtain her Associate of Applied Science Diagnostic Medical Imaging Radiography degree.

During her crisis, Bobbie learned a lot about herself. While attending groups and treatment, she completed an assessment with the therapeutic counselors. With an individualized treatment plan created for her and her husband, they immediately took part in group sessions. At the onset of her first meeting, Bobbie just sat and listened.

It wasn't long before she decided to speak up and share. As others entered the meeting, she noticed that many of them knew each other. They spoke casually in the moments before the meeting, but no one asked who she was the entire time. So, she quietly observed.

As the session began, a woman took to the podium and introduced herself. "Hi, I'm Anna and I'm an alcoholic." That was how each person introduced herself to the group. This pattern established a common identity shared by the attendees. Their addiction was an integral part of who they were and inextricably linked to their identity.

Bobbie found that only one person, obviously a newcomer, had difficulty with the self-identification: "I am an alcoholic." When this lady stood up to speak, she said, "Hi, I'm Joyce . . ." then hesitated. "I'm here because I drink too much." The other members responded in the same way they did to the long-time members, returning the greeting, "Hi Joyce!" with no judgment.

From her first meeting, Bobbie witnessed that each attendee had a story to tell. Storytelling was integral to group meetings. It is a way for attendees to share their experiences, hardships, and lessons. The idea is to create a safe community where individuals reflect upon the impact of alcohol on them personally, in their relationships, and in their careers. Common themes run throughout these stories. Many mentioned an alcoholic parent or spouse. Quite a few discussed the ways alcohol affected their jobs or their health. Many talked about God or their Higher Power.

CHAPTER TWO

FROM NASTY TO NICE

BY BOBBIE WALLACE

How important is the quality of your family life to you? As one who has struggled with alcohol addiction, it is very important to me. That is why I have made my spiritual and personal growth a priority in developing a healthy family life. By attending my support group, I have had the opportunity to reflect on my personal and professional success. I have had time to really think about my attitude towards money, responsibility, influence, and growth.

While still in treatment, I learned there was nothing wrong with any of these things. I did learn that there is something far more important that needs to come before one can attain and achieve these things. And that something is a healthy spiritual life. Having a strong spiritual life is essential because it guides your decisions. It helps you understand what you want to accomplish and how you want to grow. It's also about who you are. As you think about your life, how is your spirit faring? Are you ignoring your spirit?

I never thought a woman like me, with a *nasty* attitude, dirty and a drug-addicted life would be here today. When I was a little girl of only10 years old, I was molested by "grown men" that were friends of my mother. They told me I was ugly, black, and nasty. I then turned to drugs and alcohol to soothe all my pain for 36 Years. Then one day, I learned of the verse in Jeremiah 29:11 which says, *"For I know the thoughts that I think toward, saith the Lord, thoughts of peace, and not of evil, to give you an expected end."* When I read that verse, it changed my WORLD.

I also read another verse: "Therefore if anyone is in Christ the new creation has begun. The old is gone, the new is here (2 Corinthians 5:19, NIV). Then I began to cry out to Jesus, and He began to do wonderful work on me. I gave my life over to Christ and a new creation was born! That new creation is me. I don't drink or use drugs anymore. My attitude is no longer nasty, and I'm learning to love like Christ.

I now know that my spiritual life needs nurturing because it determines my character and perspective. It shapes the way I relate to the world and those around me. I have discovered that before I could move on to create personal success and growth, I had to first understand the value of feeding my spirit with meaning and purpose. I thank God that with the help of a great support system of caring and loving friends, I am feeding my spirit and God is blessing my family life.

A native of Chicago's West Side, **Evangelist Christel Williams** is a school clerk who was raised by a single mother. A graduate of John Marshall High School, Christel proudly serves on the school's alumni committee. She has been blessed with three daughters Arielle (32), Adrienne (30), Alexis (22), and a handsome pre-teen grandson. She has also welcomed a 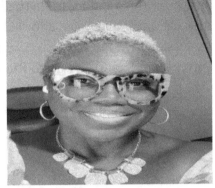 bonus daughter, Mona, whom God gave her the opportunity to pour into at an early age, and two granddaughters. Christel happens to live across the street from the school her girls attended and where she was employed as a School Clerk. Affectionately known as "Ms. Christel" to the students in and out of school, her home became a safe haven and a refuge for four other young girls.

Working in the field of education for the past 28 years, Christel was determined to survive and make the best life she could for her daughters. A veteran of Chicago Public Schools, she worked as a School Clerk for 17 years and has been employed with the Chicago Teachers Union since 2009. She always had a fight in her to help others and she used that energy in organizing the strike of 2012, prior to becoming a Union Field Representative. She won the seat as an elected officer of the union as the Recording Secretary. She also serves as a Vice President with the Illinois Federation of Teachers and works closely with the American Federation of Teachers.

As a single mother raising girls on the west side of Chicago, she knew she had to keep them busy. She supported everything they wanted to do from ballot and dance, to gymnastics, volleyball, baseball, and softball. Even now she is still supporting her middle daughter's basketball career. This daughter played basketball for the Marshall High School Lady Commandos on a state championship team under legendary coach Dorothy Gaters. After graduating from high school, she attended the University of Illinois in Champaign-

Urbana on a full scholarship where she played basketball, she has since graduated and headed off to pursue her career on a professional level. Her outstanding basketball skills and determination to be the best at the game has afforded her many opportunities to play professionally in Iceland, Germany, Dominican Republic, and currently in San Juan, Puerto Rico.

CHAPTER THREE

HAPPY AFTER THE HURT

BY CHRISTEL WILLIAMS

Oftentimes we find ourselves in situations that make us very unhappy. It may be family relationships, marriage, work environment, or something else. The list goes on and on. In any of these situations, you try to find a way to remain happy or at peace. Seeking solitude in a messed-up situation can be a challenge, even when you know God and have been raised in the church all of your life. One event or experience can trigger you to do and say some things that impact your life forever!

I have survived many situations in my life that have kept me bound for years. Not understanding them, I tended to ask the question, "Why me?" How could a woman who has been following after God's heart for as long as I have endured so much? I think of all the hard things I have been through like surviving incest, enduring robbery by gunpoint, kidnapping, rape, and searching for love in a series of bad relationships and in all the wrong places. I have been violated emotionally, psychologically, and in some cases, physically.

But it wasn't until I was able to study and meditate on God's Word that I received life changing wisdom and a better understanding of God's purpose for my life. One scripture in particular resonates in my spirit. Job 13:15 declares *"Though you slay me, yet will I trust him; but I will maintain my own ways before him."* Job was dealing with grief, loss, and disappointment as we all do on our life's journey, but you couldn't get him to say one doubtful thing to or about God. And in the midst of it all, he prayed to the Father saying: *"The Lord giveth, and he taketh away; blessed be the name of the Lord"* (Job 1:21).

Be encouraged when you're going through difficult situations and be willing to let things go! Replace them with the fruits of the Spirit: *love, joy, peace, forbearance, kindness, goodness and faithfulness* (Galatians 5:22-23). Ponder on these attributes for a second. Love when it's hard to love; be joyful and excited about what's to come; seek tranquility; have patience, self-control, and tolerance; be kind when they are mean to you; be virtuous and practice good morals; and most of all, remain faithful until the end. I found that by practicing these principles, I can smile, I can survive, I'm winning again, and I am happy in my hurt!

Psalm 84:11 NIV assures us that *"The Lord God is a sun and shield; the Lord bestows favor and honor; no good thing will He withhold from those who seek him!* I took that word and ran with it. I began to apply it to everything I thought I had lost. Now I take comfort in the promise of Job 8:7. Although my start was small, my latter would be greater than my past!

Lisa Freeney is a woman of great strength and a leader at American Airlines for the past 33+ years. She has been married for twenty-nine years to an amazing man who encourages her to be her best self at all costs. This gracious 53 yrs. old is the mother of three beautiful, living children. It's evident whenever you greet her that she loves the Lord with all her heart.

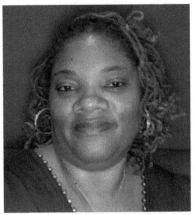

Born and raised in Chicago, Lisa loves and supports her Pastors, Leroy & Lady Katie Elliot, and her New Greater St John CMBC family. They have truly challenged her to follow and pursue her dreams on every level.

An amazing sister and friend, Lisa is one of the Co-Founders of #Gonegirl Women Empowerment Group Chicago, an organization which packs power! She is a lover of shopping and great entertainment. At this point in her life, she believes it is time for her husband and her to live their best lives. Lisa recognizes there are times in life when God creates the stage for His children to share their heart with whomever is in need. She is confident that God can count on her because as she says, "I'm the daughter of A King".

CHAPTER FOUR

SPEAK TO ME
(WORDS FROM GOD)
BY LISA FREENEY

*Whether it be good, or whether it be evil, we will obey the
voice of the Lord our God, to whom we send thee; that it may be
well with us, when we obey the voice of the Lord our God.*
Jeremiah 42:6 KJV

I always used to wonder why my life was such a mess. I typically
went about my day doing my own thing until I found out the hard
way that I can't do anything without God's word and His guidance.
There were so many times I didn't hear the voice of God speaking to
me. I did things, thought things, went places that I had no business
going to, and said things I never should have said because I was not
listening to God's voice.

When I did hear God speaking to me, it was when I was most still
in my quiet time. For so long I could not hear Him at all because of my
sinful and busy life. But God is always there when I need Him and
when I read His Word. Psalm 119:105 KJV confirms that *"Thy word is a
lamp unto my feet and a light unto my path."* When I do read the Bible, He
speaks to my heart and I feel the peace of God knowing that He won't
lead me astray. He promises me in Psalm 119:2 KJV that *"Blessed are they
that keep his testimonies and that seek him with the whole heart."*

Whenever you want to hear from God, get in a quiet, still place
and listen. He will speak to you through His Word. In Psalm 119:11
(KJV) we read, *"Thy word have I hid in my heart that I might not sin against*

thee." When I read my Bible, God gives me a word to get through each day. He will give you revelation in His Word to lift your spirit and comfort you when you need it too. Psalm 121:1 KJV encourages us to seek the Lord's help: *"I will lift up mine eyes unto the hills from whence cometh my help, my help cometh from the Lord which made heaven earth."*

Today is a good day to listen for the voice of the Lord. Will you say, "Speak to me, God!"?

Pastor Sabrina M. Hazzard has a heart and a zeal for women who are hurting. God has given Pastor Sabrina such a grace to minister to women from every walk of life. Even though she has many roles such as wife, mother, and friend, she is very passionate about the spiritual wholeness and well-being of women. Pastor Sabrina is passionate about seeing women who have suffered brokenness due to trauma and life's

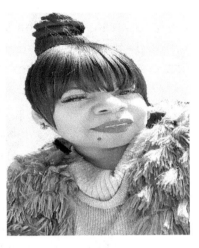

challenges be made whole, healed, and restored. God told her, "Your mess is going to be your masterpiece for others. So, whatever you have gone through, is not just for you. It's also for someone else to see that I'm the same God that can also bring them through. I will bring them out by the power of the many testimonies you have experienced in your own life." God has made it possible for Pastor Sabrina to have her own women's study group entitled, "Women Living 2 Please the Lord." It is in this group where the process begins and where lives are continually changed.

As a means of continued fellowship, strengthening, unification, and bonding with the women of Faithworld Family Worship Center, Pastor Sabrina pours into the women through women's fellowships. These intimate social gatherings are always filled with good fun and great food! The fellowships are up close and personal and allow the women of FFWC to not only get to know Pastor Sabrina, but to also bond with one another as well.

Women of War, Armed & Dangerous, birthed the monthly overnight spiritual weekend retreats, fellowship gatherings, and daily discussion groups for women by utilizing prayer conference calls, and social media forums like GroupMe chat, Zoom, and Facebook. These forums are also a viable means by which Pastor Sabrina's vision of encouraging and imparting into women, remains alive and operative.

Whether the gatherings take place at venues such as Panera Bread or the Marriott Residence Inn Suites, Pastor Sabrina is the consummate spiritual mother and teacher! She loves good books, great conversations, and good healthy food!

FFWC women are continuously being fed spiritually and being taught to live authentic, healthy, and holy lives for God! In these intimate group settings, FFWC's women's ministry book club was launched. Pastor Sabrina selects various books, three to four times annually, to be read as a group and discussed on a weekly basis.

Outside of her ministerial passions, she is a member of The Top Ladies of Distinction, Incorporated (TLOD), Midway Chicago Chapter. TLOD is a humanitarian organization which highlights women, seniors, top teens, community beautification, and community partnerships. In 2014, she was honored by TLOD with the Women Empowering Women Community Award, for her outstanding work and dedication to uplifting women in the Chicagoland area.

Healthy living and healthy loving are Pastor Sabrina's passions! She is elated to be married to her true Boaz, Terrence Dexter Hazzard, and is the proud mother of Terrence Dexter Jr., Paradeja Chivelea, Tyler David, and Taylor Derrion.

CHAPTER FIVE

PAIN 2 POWER

BY PASTOR SABRINA M. HAZZARD

Dear Diary,

God has a way of testing your strength in weak moments. He has a way of testing your faith during times of uncertainty. He has a way of making you question His hand on your life during the darkest hours of your life. God, what happened? What did I do to deserve this? Where are you? I needed you YESTERDAY!

If you haven't had these moments yet, they're coming! This is not to scare you, but it's to inform you that before you can get to your next level, before you can grow in your faith, and before you can mature in your gift, there will be a TEST! I've had many tests in my life. However, the test that I feel was a true turning point in my faith and in my relationship with God, was given to me in October 2020! It was a test that I will NEVER FORGET!

In October 2020, I was invited to a women's conference. Due to the global Covid-19 pandemic, I had not been outside since March 2020, so I wanted to make sure that I didn't move prematurely. I had to make sure the health and safety of my family was my first priority. I definitely didn't want to be presumptuous in my decision to attend the conference. The keynote speaker was one that I followed for some time, and I felt that this was my only chance to see her in person. Seeing her name on the ticket had me so excited! I was sure she would have a word for me at that conference. With hesitation and much prayer, I decided to attend.

As I often do, I decided to invite a few ladies that lived near the venue. They were just as excited as I was to attend the conference.

They bought their tickets and beat me there! As I was preparing to go to the conference, EVERYTHING was going wrong! I lost my car keys. I didn't know what to wear. I needed to be a wife and Mom all at once, and I still hadn't found my car keys. Looking back, I wonder if it could have been God trying to get me to calm down and listen? But why would God want me to miss an encounter that I felt I needed?

After being on lockdown since March, I was desperate for a breath of fresh air after what felt like 10 months. So, of course, I thought the devil was trying to keep me from receiving a word from the Lord. That's another point I want to make. We sometimes think when everything is in shambles, it must be the enemy trying to distract us. Could it be God saying, "Have a seat and listen to what I'm trying to tell you"?

After all of the setbacks, we finally found the keys, loaded up, and hit the road. Upon our arrival, they checked our temperatures as promised, and it appeared that the majority of the conference participants were wearing masks. I found the group I had invited, and we all sat in a section with only about 4 other people who were not a part of our group. We never removed our masks. I knew my group didn't play about wearing their masks and keeping their hands clean. I made sure I followed all of the CDC regulations. I wore my mask, washed my hands, and whatever else they recommended. The conference was awesome! My group and I enjoyed the speaker.

Fast forward to the end of the day. I immediately started feeling sick. At first, I thought it was all in my mind, but two days later it hit me like a ton of bricks. I was sick with Covid. That dreadful sickness I had seen take many loved ones out had now hit me! I was devastated. Not only was I sick, but the group of ladies who went with me also had tested positive for Covid-19. Immediately, I began to question God. "God, how?" "God, why?" "God, why me?" This is where the fight started, both physically and spiritually.

I became weaker by the minute. I had never been this sick in my entire life. Even after giving birth three times, nothing compared to the awful pain I was in. The nights were the worst. I literally had the death angel visit me, and I was being tormented both day and night. I could hear an audible voice saying that I wouldn't make it through the week. The enemy wanted me dead! He wanted my faith to end. He wanted my strength to be gone. If it weren't for my family, I would have given up. My baby boy, Taylor, played a recording of scriptures all day, every day. He would hold my hand and ask, "Mom, are you ok?" Sometimes I didn't have the strength to respond. I would just nod. My husband would come and pray. He offered me all kinds of home remedies.

Then there was Tyler who could hardly stomach seeing me sick and in so much pain. One day I remember my family sitting at the edge of my bed. They all grabbed hands and began to praise and shout. That's so important. In your darkest and weakest moment, you have to make sure the people around you don't give up until they see you back and stronger than ever. I mustered up enough strength and just lifted my hands. At that moment, I knew I had to praise my way out of this.

Weak and full of doubt, I began to command healing to me as my measure. I told God I wasn't ready to die. I told Him how much my family needed me and that I still had much ministry to fulfill. I begin to ask God to take away any unforgiveness that I had hidden in my heart. Please take away any bitterness, strife, etc. because those spirits can cause sickness like cancer or even anxiety. After I sought God sincerely, I mean truly repented and praised my way through, I felt my symptoms leaving supernaturally. I was able to take my vitamins and my color started coming back. It was in my weakest hours that I felt God's presence. My faith grew and my love for my family, friends and even life was restored. My pain gave me POWER!! My weakness strengthened me. My trust in God was stronger than ever because He became my Healer, Physician, and Restorer.

God will RESTORE you!

Valante Maria is the founder of the byDesign Network. She is a storyteller who incorporates the use of digital media to empower people to stir up their God-given gifts and live life according to divine purpose. Her body of work spans across literary, audio, and visual platforms. As executive producer of The Sanctuary Academy YouTube channel, Valante has built an audience of over 1.3 million people globally. In 2021, she launched the "Life Design Studio," 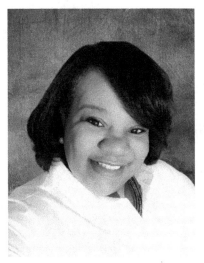 where she facilitates online courses and provides faith coaching services. Valante is a TEDx organizer and active TED (TED Talks) member, currently hosting monthly TED Circles. She is a Subject Matter Expert for SCORE & the SBA where she conducts YouTube training sessions. Valante is a true servant leader who has committed her life to cultivating humanity.

CHAPTER SIX

STUCK IN THE MIDDLE

BY VALANTE MARIA

As a single mother, my priority has always been to provide the absolute best quality of life for my daughter. I tried to compensate for the lack of a father present in the home by exposing her to positive influences and extraordinary life experiences. Between working and spending time with her, there was very little time left for me. I felt like this is what motherhood was all about. Once my daughter made it to her sophomore year of high school, I thought that I would be able to "breathe" a little. Just when I thought I could finally reclaim some time for myself, my mother started to display signs of the onset of Dementia. I felt trapped in the middle of caring for a child and my parents. Between my parents and my daughter, there was always something that needed to be done. When there was a quiet moment, I would be so exhausted. I felt unable to do anything. Sometimes I would literally just sit and stare into space.

I had always planned to be there to care for my parents as they aged because they gave me such an amazing childhood. But, I was not prepared for my mother's decline. I watched her deteriorate before my very eyes daily. I distinctly remember the day I realized that we would never go shopping again, never go to lunch again, never go to church together again, and never take a trip together again. This stress of my mother's condition distracted me from my role as a parent. The next thing I knew, my daughter was in crisis. She didn't want to confide in me because she could see that I was overwhelmed. Her life began to spiral out of control. I felt like I was losing the only thing that truly mattered to me--my family!

For 5 years, I struggled to hold everything and everybody together. There were days when I was too tired to even eat. Just to have a moment of peace, I would cook dinner and go sit quietly alone while everyone else ate. I no longer had a life and I dreaded waking up in the mornings. I didn't even realize I had completely lost myself. Without even realizing it, I had plunged into a state of depression and grief. It got to a point where I crashed. I was completely depleted and could do nothing. Everything seemed to be falling down around me.

That's when I gave it to God. There was one thing I learned from my mother that pulled me through. She taught me how to fast and pray. From watching her example, I learned how to talk to God and more importantly, to listen to God. He showed me that I wasn't stuck in the middle. I decided to put myself in the middle of His business instead. We are all God's children--my parents, my daughter, and me. It was never my assignment to take care of us. My assignment was to trust God to take care of us. Feeling lost comes from not following God. Feeling overwhelmed comes from not trusting God.

Since then, I've learned that there will never be time for me unless I make time for myself. I will never get those 5 years of my life back. I'm not trying to make up for lost time. I'm not worried about the future either. I've learned to be present and to enjoy the moment. I put myself on my calendar. If I don't show up for me, there will be no me to show up for anyone else. I was really never taking care of anyone, including myself, anyway. It was always God all along.

Easter Coleman is one of ten children who came from humble beginnings and raised in the Cabrini Green Projects of Chicago. Her passion for cooking began early with her preparing food on her barbecue grill outside the building where she lived at 929 N Hudson in Chicago.

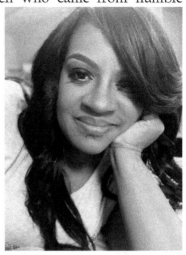

Easter's amazing flavors were new and very tasty to her community and passersby. Everyone who ate her dishes loved them. They even craved her cooking on a daily basis. Soon Easter began to realize she had a real gift to satisfy the taste buds of others with her culinary gift. After this revelation, Easter began to wholeheartedly pursue cooking, sharing her recipes and ideas with any and everyone who asked for her help. Since she was giving so much of her time to cooking, she let her gift make room for her. As a single mom of eight children, she realized she could use her skills to generate revenue for her family.

Today Easter has been in the culinary industry for more than twenty years. During her culinary adventures she has evolved in many ways and reached new milestones. She has been a certified ServSafe instructor for 5 years. She has also obtained a City Of Chicago Shared Kitchen License and started her own catering business. One particularly exciting event in Easter's culinary adventure was the grand opening of her restaurant in Gary, Indiana in September 2020!

The inspiration for her business' name, "Easter's Cuisine" came from her desire to infuse love into every dish she creates for the world. Healthy eating became her focus when her grandmother (Maude Dobbs) died due to high blood pressure, kidney dysfunction, congestive heart failure, and lung disease.

Now Easter is ready to adapt to the evolving trends of the culinary arts. She has refined her skills and pursued extra education by becoming a graduate of Washburne Culinary & Hospitality Institute. As a certified Chef, Easter is focused and highly motivated. She has established a non-profit organization to support and provide educational activities to enhance and transform the lives of disadvantaged youth and young adults. The goal of the program is to help prevent crime within neighborhoods through trade and business instruction. She hopes to combat prodigal behaviors in the community as well. Easter plans to share her passion and skills through catering, meal prep, healthy eating workshops, cooking demos, and education.

CHAPTER SEVEN

FORGET WHAT YOU HEARD, GIRL! YOU ARE WORTH IT! "SELF-WORTH"

BY EASTER COLEMAN

The simple pleasures of life were hard to obtain growing up in the Cabrini Green housing project. As a young, short-haired black girl, I thought I was just a 1 on a scale of 10. Already darker than most children and ugly in my mind, you could say I held a negative mental image of myself. While in this frame of mind, the experience of incest and molestation became all too real for this ugly black girl. Growing up just happened and I soon gave birth to children.

Even after becoming a mom, I still felt like a little, ugly, black girl on the inside. I was constantly trying to find my worth. It was not an easy process. Dealing with what happened to me, who did it, and forgiving yourself were all the puzzle pieces that spoke the loudest. But as India Arie would say, there is hope!

I learned through my personal experience with God that taking the time to really allow Him to heal me from the inside out was the beginning of having life for real. One scripture which helped me to believe when I didn't understand my value was Psalms 134:14: *"I will praise thee, for I am fearfully and wonderfully made marvelous are your works and that my soul knows it well."* This scripture was the catalyst for my deliverance. With tears in my eyes and disbelief of the scripture in my heart, I rehearsed it daily until it happened--the breaking of day! I spoke *"those things that are not as though they were"* (Romans 4:17).

Then, that spirit broke off me and I was "NO MORE SAD" (1 Samuel 1:18). With man (me myself & I) this was impossible; but, oh the word of God gave me a very different perception! Matthew 19:26 declares that God specializes in the impossible. So, I say to YOU who are reading this, WHATEVER your issue may be that is speaking louder in your life than God, help yourself to drown out the noise by first believing, then repeating until God's word until it gets deep in your spirit. Know that the change you desire is a work for God. He can and will handle you as perfectly as you are. Be happy and glow up honey because it's going to happen for you just like it did for me (Philippians 1:6). Love you to pieces because you are just the BOMB.com baby!

Public Speaker. Author. Publisher. Singer/Songwriter. Entrepreneur. **Deirdre Cunningham,** affectionately known as Lady C, is a faithful, compassionate and affectionate mother of 5, the wife of Kevin (since 1994), a daughter, sister, friend and confidante to many.

Lady C relentlessly serves in ministry as Executive Pastor alongside her husband, Kevin Cunningham, Senior Pastor, at The Transformation Center Chicago. Their focus in ministry and life is to always demonstrate the love of God, inspire faith in God, and reconcile the lost to God.

Lady C is passionate about being transparent in all she does because she believes her experiences allow her to counsel others and encourage them to learn and grow. She loves to implement strategies and concepts which provide those she serves the best opportunities to live, thrive, and soar. An exemplary leader and devout woman of virtue, she is focused on fulfilling her life's purpose to bring healing to as many women as possible before leaving earth.

CHAPTER EIGHT

DON'T RACE, JUST RUN

BY DEIRDRE CUNNINGHAM

I felt as if I would never be able to catch up. Everyone else seemed to be getting things done. Doors seemed to be opening for them so quickly. As soon as I thought I was in a stride, I would receive a notification and see something new and exciting happening for them yet again.

I immediately and intensely started talking to the Lord about all these people who were receiving theirs while I struggled to get mine. *What am I doing wrong? What am I not doing that I should be doing? Have I totally missed something?* I thought, *Lord, you told me that this is my turn and my season. What happened to all of that which you promised me?*

This dialogue from me to the Lord continued for about 8 days. Then, the Lord began to speak to me. He started to show me what I was really feeling inside. He started to reveal to me that my innermost feelings were blocking my progress, not anything around me. I had lost confidence in my husband, my children, my church, myself, and ultimately, the Lord. I fully embraced this truth as the Lord spoke sternly, but lovingly to my heart. I was so ashamed that I had allowed myself to get so far off track.

That's when I realized how I was ogling others who seemed impressive to me. I should have merely observed them, taken note of the good qualities that I saw, and made adjustments to my own life where improvements were needed, all the while continuing to pursue my niche.

What had happened was that I had become secretly doubtful of myself. As a result, I had begun to place confidence in others by trying to emulate them. If someone had a successful event, I would try to tweak it enough to call it mine and then try to replicate it. If someone changed and had a strong presence from head to toe, I tried to remake myself to have the same outside effect.

Once I completed my conversation with the Lord, I received wisdom for the 5-Pillar Principle that I now teach to women in a course called Simply ME. This principle also sets the new course for my life and establishes my purpose for living to bring healing to as many women as possible before leaving this earth.

Now, I have a clear and steady path and direction for accomplishing my divine purpose. As the saying goes, I am now comfortable in my own skin. I am confident and keep a steady gait toward my life goals. There is no greater joy than this!

How did this happen? I'm so glad you asked. I stopped competing with those that I secretly admired and began living my best self as God had originally intended and designed. That is what I mean when I say, "Just Run." Stop looking around and bear down and do what is expected and what you have the ability to do. Once you get these principles in your innermost being, you too will stop the Race and start your Run.

Tracey E Gordon has a passion to serve, help, lift, and encourage little girls, young women, and women who have been abused and mistreated. Her ministry is to the fragmented and broken-hearted. She wants people to see how perfectly fitted they are designed for GOD'S divine purpose.

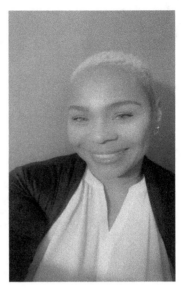

Tracey has been at the Chicago Transit Authority for twenty-eight years. When not serving people, she loves traveling, shopping, pampering, and spending time with family and friends. Tracey is married to Allen C Gordon Jr, and has two daughters Megan (24 years, and Trinity (14 years).

Contact Information
Email tracey_gordon3@yahoo.com
Facebook pumpkingt3
Facebook Tracey Gordon (Tracey E Ross)

CHAPTER NINE

BROKEN BUT NOT SHATTERED

BY TRACEY GORDON

And so, dear brothers and sisters,[a] I plead with you to give your bodies to God because of all he has done for you. Let them be a living and holy sacrifice—the kind he will find acceptable. This is truly the way to worship him. 2 Don't copy the behavior and customs of this world, but let God transform you into a new person by changing the way you think. Then you will learn to know God's will for you, which is good and pleasing and perfect. Romans 12:1-2 NLT

I'm broken but I'm not shattered; I'm broken but not shattered beyond repair. I'm broken but GOD mended the pieces back together for His Glory and a part of His Story within my story.

So, what caused my brokenness? When I was a young child, a more fragmented and broken person abused me and caused me to become broken. She violated me by doing and making me do things to her that no child should do. For 3 years, this woman violated and then rejected me. Rejection opened my spirit up to some very vile and lustful thoughts, ideas, and imaginations for most of my teen and young adult years.

At the age of 13, I was baptized and accepted God in my life. I struggled with how God could love this crazy, tormented, and filthy little girl with all these issues. I received the Holy Spirit and the gift of speaking in tongues at age 18. But, this didn't change my bad behavior; I was out of control.

Then in 2003, God started my DELIVERANCE process. Yes, I was still broken, but I wasn't shattered beyond repair. The scriptures that fed my soul and brought me back at that time were. Romans 12:1-2, Romans 8:1, James 1:14, Colossians 3:5, 1 John 2:16, and Galatians 6:8. These scriptures brought me through.

It's a journey and a daily process to stay free, but God delivered me! He silenced the questions in my head, and I learned to silence the enemy from talking to me in my members. I stopped the identity questioning, the masturbation, pornography, and adultery which were not faithful to GOD and my spouse.

I'm broken, but not shattered, because GOD loves me. He saw my beginning from my end and still shines His glorious reflections through all my broken pieces.

Be encouraged. Your BROKENNESS is for a greater purpose. Be healed and not shattered. Because God created you, He knows your strength and what you can bear. He knows you and formed you, He knows what you can endure. Because His Spirit is moving in you, He knows how far you can be pushed.

God reassured and reminded me of His big picture view of my life. He spoke to my heart: "You ran from me when I pushed, but you always returned to me because I was calling from the depths of your heart. I drew you with my love because you are mine. Because, I knew that rejection from the womb would change your views from the start, I constructed a fortress around you to sustain the blows. Because I knew abuse would try to change your identity, I made you with a desire to always come and find me."

"Because I'm your Father, your Protector, your Sustainer, and your Redeemer I came and found you where you were and recused you. I cleansed you from the depths of sin's stain, gave you a new heart, and a new identity. I know what I put in you, and I knew you could stand because you're My child and I've been with you always."

When I was molested as a young girl, there was no one there to take the pain away. When I was raped, there was no one to talk to. When I was pregnant, there was no one to hold my hand. But one day when I was on my way to swallow those pills, I heard Your voice and felt Your presence. The Holy Spirit whispered, "I Love you and you're mine. I created you to be mine. I know things have happened to you but that wasn't my plan for you."

GOD is faithful and always on time. Never turn your back on GOD for His Word and His plan is always on time. GOD is just and He will keep you through your storms. Just trust and believe it's not by your power or strength that you will overcome the obstacles. It was the indwelling Spirit that will bring you through. So, recover from your places of pain. God can heal you and move you to the other side of pain.

Chaplain LaTonya Herron is the mother of 2 beautiful children and grandmother of 2 amazing granddaughters. She loves loving on GOD. Her career spans over 30 years at American Airlines where she served as an EAP Rep for Twu Org. This speaks volumes of her compassion and hunger to succeed.

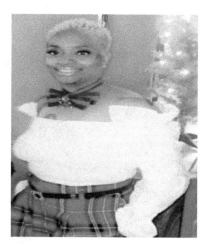

LaTonya loves to decorate and beautify homes. Making decor come to life is quite fulfilling for her. In her spare time, she is an adamant reader and traveler.

As LaTonya continues to mature in the things of GOD, her passion for loving people the right way grows. If you only knew her story you would know that LaTonya is a survivor and she doesn't take that for granted. She's pegged as an encourager and is always sharing with others how God helps you to fulfill being the best you can be.

Her passions include feeding and clothing the homeless, which she has done now for over 25 years. Additionally, LaTonya helps to build grass roots in the ministry so they can get a great start. Her accomplishments include serving as Co-Founder of OneSister2Another Media & #Gonegirl Women Empowerment Group of Chicago IL, both led by Pastor Angela Johnson. LaTonya is God's girl and you better know it.

CHAPTER TEN

SHATTERED PIECES, YET I RISE!

BY CHAPLAIN LATONYA SHERRIA HERRON

"You may shoot me with your words, you may cut me with your eyes, you may kill me with your hatefulness, but still, like air, I'll rise. I rise! I rise!" Maya Angelou

I am laying in my bed wondering, *Do I want to fix myself some breakfast, read my Bible, grab my phone and gossip with my girls, or get up and go slash my husband's tires for something I'm still holding a grudge about.*

As I lay there contemplating, I knew I was not dealing with the real issue. I needed to come face to face with my brokenness and pain. Here I was in my 3rd marriage and once again getting a divorce. I couldn't hide behind the fake smiles anymore. I couldn't keep lying to my family and friends telling them I'm alright. My true issue was ME. How could God love someone so messed up like me? I am broken into so many pieces, stuck in dysfunction, and crushed mentally beyond repair. I was ashamed. I could not tell anyone how I truly felt. I was worried about what people were going to say! Who would understand this craziness?

In this dark place, I couldn't even hear God's voice anymore. I cried out, "It's me again God. GOD WHERE ARE YOU?" I fell to my knees all alone and in agony. "God, I have no one BUT YOU!"

Then in all this madness and chaos, I hear a small whisper. And God said to me, *"My grace is sufficient for you, for my strength is made perfect in your weaknesses* (2 Corinthians 12:9).*"*

I was able to RISE despite the shame and embarrassment. I could RISE from the brokenness and pain. I finally could RISE to become the Mighty Woman of God I'm called to. In my position of worship, God taught me in my valley, my low place! (Psalm 23:4).

Now I can say, I am loved! I am valuable! I am strong. Now, I RISE!

Melissa Walls is a believer that God is real. She also believes that she has been given the grace to lead. At 54 years old she has been in Aviation for over thirty-two years with American Airlines at O'hare International Airport in Chicago.

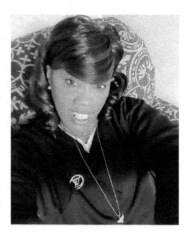

She is married to Michael A Walls and through their amazing union they have five children, three of her own and two bonus kids. Their children include three daughters and two sons: Davon R Ferguson, Kailynn M Ferguson, Rakeeya R Walls, Mykah A Walls and Darius H Ferguson. Melissa is also blessed to have four grandkids.

In addition to being a wife, mother and grandmother, this woman of God is a daughter, sister, and a friend to many. She knows that her walk with God is not always easy, but she refuses to give up on Him in any way shape or form. Today she is truly proud of herself as she continues to walk by faith and not give up no matter what she's going through in her day-to-day challenges. She is a woman who continues to trust God.

CHAPTER ELEVEN

REFUSE TO LOSE IN YOUR LOSS
MY GRIEF: GOD' BURDEN

BY MELISSA S WALLS

For this is how God loved the world: He gave[a] his one and only Son, so that everyone who believes in him will not perish but have eternal life. St. John 3:16 NLT

"Wow, I'm so grateful, thankful, and blessed!" That's how I woke up this morning. Praise God! I woke up feeling refreshed and renewed. This is no time for feeling down, weeping and crying! It's time to show God I appreciate Him!

As I was sitting and thinking about the past 2 years, I knew they had really been rough for me. First, my son passed. I struggled with the fact that my own brother killed my son. Then my husband left me for 3 months and I went back to work and injured my back. Now as I'm writing, I have Covid 19. I have every reason to doubt God, right? But I decided that through it all, I would not! God never left me, and He is still here walking with me through it all!

God is great even when we turn our backs on him. Even when we doubt Him, He is still there with open arms ready to welcome us back when we finally come to our senses.

"Listen," I told myself, "You will die in this mess unless you get up, change your mindset, and decide that you are going to live".

My faith has gotten so strong now that I will never doubt Our Abba Father anymore. I always knew God was real, but I had sat in self-pity feeling hurt, mad, and sorry for myself. Now God is showing me that I am a chosen one. I can share with others a positive word that when you're down and out, God will deliver you. I'm chosen to share goodness about who He is. Life isn't easy all the time. We will go through situations, yet He's always right there with us to fight our battles. We just have to believe and trust Him.

We do have to put in the work, but God gives us the tools to be prepared at all times. We have to put on the full armor of God and be prepared to fight the battle. I decided to decree "I will win, and God will get the glory no matter what!"

We can't be scared when we walk with God, nor should we be living in fear when He promises not to ever leave us nor forsake us. He has proven to me that He's worthy of my trust. I am so glad that God has never given up on me, even when I gave up on myself. What a Mighty God we serve. Praise the Lord! Amen! Hallelujah! This is my story. This is my testimony.

Sabrina Roosevelt is a wife and mother. She was born and raised on the west side of Chicago where she not only overcame drug use, but also the life of a drug dealer. Sabrina has claimed victory over a lifestyle of drugs, sexual and physical abuse, incarceration, violence, sexual confusion, and attempted suicide. She now dedicates her life to seeing women healed, delivered, and made whole.

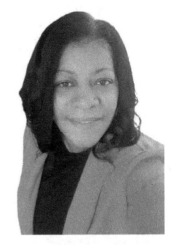

As a prophetic voice and intercessor, she labors to see the broken places of women and young adults healed, delivered, and set free. Sabrina does this by sharing her testimony of how God delivered her from shame, guilt, and condemnation. She speaks of the once broken places of her life and shares her story to help others.

She also uses her business, *Paraklesis Designs*, to express her passion, love, and gift of encouragement to express the heart of God. Many have come to accept Christ into their lives and have been delivered from places of hopelessness and suicidal thoughts due to her willingness to partner with God by sharing her heart of compassion. Sabrina prayerfully intercedes for others. She encourages them to receive the will of God for their lives and resist the forces of the enemy that hold them back. Sabrina now resides in Janesville, Wisconsin with her husband Jukoda Roosevelt. Together they attend Northside Christian Assembly.

Sabrinaroosevelt709@gmail.com
(Facebook) Sabrina Roosevelt
(Clubhouse) @sabrina_warrior
(Instagram) heart_intercessor

CHAPTER TWELVE

I'M COMING OUT!

BY SABRINA ROOSEVELT

43 When he had said this, Jesus called in a loud voice, "Lazarus, come out!"
44 The dead man came out, his hands and feet wrapped with strips of linen, and a
cloth around his face. Jesus said to them, "Take off the grave clothes and let him
go."
John 11:43-44

As a child, I dealt with the pain of rejection and molestation. As I grew older, I had no idea the impact it would have on my life. I turned to drugs and sex at a very tender age to mask the eternal pain of being taken advantage of and the impact of family rejection. The consequences led me to a life that I was not prepared for. As I progressed in my drug use, it led to several incarcerations, being committed to a drug treatment facility, having several reinstated probations, disconnection from my children, a terrifying abusive relationship that almost killed me, and eventually, attempted suicide. Drugs took me farther than I wanted to go, kept me longer than I wanted to stay, and cost me more than I was willing to pay.

As I sit here writing this devotional, my heart is thinking of you, the reader. I am thinking of how you are being led by God just like I was. It is not by chance that you are reading a small, but profound, portion of my story. It is not by chance that the Lord allowed me to write it. This is an intentional moment, a Kairos moment in time that has been established before you were formed in your mother's womb. THIS IS YOUR EXODUS! This is your appointment to come out of all the things that have wounded you. This is your time to come out of that grave of your past and rid yourself of the stench that constantly reminds you of an open wound.

Perhaps your trauma isn't rejection or molestation. In every case, the road to recovery, healing, and wholeness is the same. Jesus is the way, the truth, and the life. He came so that we would have life and have it more abundantly (healed and whole). Your healing has already been made available through the work of the cross. As God draws you, which I believe He's doing right now as you read this devotional, you can yield to what the Holy Spirit is saying to you. Not only will you come out, but you'll be in a position to help someone else come out of their grave. You see, our stories help one another. It helps to strengthen and encourage one another. Better yet, our journey and story of God's power to heal, positions us to partner with Him in assisting to heal and or deliver our sister. With that being said, did you know that someone is waiting on you to come out so you can help them out?

As you begin to acknowledge where you are and ask God to come into your place of brokenness, He will begin to take you on a journey of healing. In this journey you will experience His presence like never before. He will show you the truth of who you are and will eradicate every lie that the enemy has spoken over you and concerning your future.

Today is your day to move towards healing and wholeness. Speak and declare what the Lord reveals to you. Speak His Word and watch those words be made manifest in your life.

This is your EXODUS! Be encouraged for the Lord your God is not only with you, but He's leading and guiding you into places that go beyond your human reasoning. I can hear Him calling you, can't you hear Him? Answer Him and He will reveal Himself to you. He will take you into places of intimacy with Him that will lead and guide you into total freedom.

LaShawn Wallace is a wife, friend, mentor, award-winning creative educator, and union organizer with over 34 years of experience. She utilizes her deep spiritual faith and knowledge as a catalyst to promote positive change in individuals and community settings.

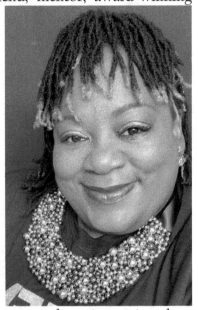

She grew up on the west side of Chicago and extracts from her experiences to assist those in need as an author, life coach, and everyday theologian. She draws from her deeply personal experiences in the classroom, boardroom, and church pews to integrate a joyful and solemn analysis of God's grace that guides tortuous lives into miraculous transformations.

A friend to everyone she meets, LaShawn uses her experiences and wisdom accumulated from the trenches of life to share the testimony of countless women encouraged in faith and hope to resolve painful situations and reach brighter horizons.

CHAPTER THIRTEEN

YOUR INCREASE AND YOUR DESIRES FROM GOD ARE ALL ABOUT WHAT YOU PUT INTO PRACTICE

BY LASHAWN WALLACE

I had to learn how to put into practice what I wanted from God, so that He could bring the increase in my life! I grew up in the church and when I was 22, I got married. In the beginning all was well and we were so much in love. I always prayed, fasted, and believed God's word over my life. But when things started to go bad within my marriage, I found myself crying many days and nights and asking the Lord, why? I lived holy, I fasted, and prayed. After some time, I decided to leave my marriage. I felt unloved and unwanted and so I took matters into my own hands. Not long after being separated from my husband, I began to take a more serious look at God after I had been praying and fasting for answers. I resolved to know His Word and learn His Word as final authority.

The scripture that came to me was James 2:17 KJV which says, "*Faith without works is dead.*" God was letting me know that I had to start taking steps towards the things I wanted Him to increase in my life. From the day I began to put in practice the Word of God, I saw an increase in my commitment to Him and to myself regarding all the things I desired for Him to do for me and all that I aspired to do.

God allowed His Word to encourage me and give me a reason for living. I saw things with heaven's eyes about what I desired in life. My desire was to be a God-fearing wife, an amazing mom, and leader.

Lastly, I desired that God's Word would cause me to increase, direct me, and protect me from myself. I'm a living witness today that He will watch over His Word to perform it.

Yolanda Carter is a woman of courage and strength who turned her pain to purpose. Her life proves that no matter how bad it may look, you can make it. Her life is necessary because test after test, still she rises. Yolanda's story of surviving domestic violence has been featured on WGN-TV. She has decided to live so she rises up early to bless God daily for all He has brought her through.

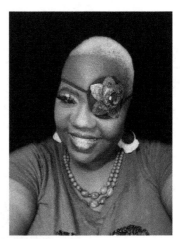

A strong and resilient woman, Yolanda shares her story globally because she refuses to be silent any longer. The mother of 5 children (3 boys and 2 girls) ranging from 22 to 36, she is also blessed with 10 grandchildren. She often says there were times she didn't think she would live to see her children grow up and become adults. But God didn't suffer it to be so. He brought her out of that situation. Today her story is being broadcast all over the globe via her first book, **One Eyewitness, Breaking The Silence Of Domestic Violence.**

Yolanda's life is one of triumph and enormous victories. She has pressed through some challenges that have caused her to recover on all levels. She says that she has her joy back. She can see clearer now and has a goal of starting a recovery home where women who suffer in silence can be free to restart their lives free of fear. She believes it is of utmost importance that women and children who experience any type of violence know that they are loved and there is help.

CHAPTER FOURTEEN

BEAUTY FOR MY ASHES

BY YOLANDA CARTER

On the morning of March 22, 2016, my life changed forever! After falling asleep that night, I was suddenly awakened by my baby boy who was shaking me trying to get my attention. He was very confused about what was going on. Meanwhile, I was going in and out of consciousness. I could hear faint sounds of sirens. When I finally came through, I discovered that my partner had tried to take my life while I was asleep. He had beaten me with a hammer and left me to die in a pool of blood.

But thank God, I survived although I had suffered severe physical damage and mental scars. Domestic violence is real. One out of three women and one out of seven men will be affected by domestic violence in their lifetime. I never thought this would ever happen to me. At one time, I thought I had everything under control. I had never expected my knight in shining armor to treat me this way. How could this happen?

When you suffer domestic violence, never think it's your fault because it's not. And domestic violence is not only black eyes and bruises. This cycle of abuse is also mental, emotional, verbal, psychological, financial, and spiritual. Always pay attention to the red flags and warning signs. If only I had paid attention. The writing was on the wall, but I ignored it. Remember there's always a warning before action!! I am motivated to warn others through sharing my story and how it impacted my family.

Yes, it was very traumatizing for my son to find me that way. It was like a horror flick out of a movie. My situation was touch and go, but God stayed in the midst of it and shielded me. The initial shock came of when they told me that they had to remove my left eye. At first, I didn't have any emotions and didn't know what was going on. A metal plate was placed in my skull to save my life. So much damage had been done I didn't know what to think.

All I knew was that I wanted to live. After all this, I'm now starting to recover and rebuild my life! I had to go through therapy to learn how to cope and live my new normal without being ashamed or embarrassed. I am not giving up. I speak my truth to help others. My God I serve didn't bring me this far to leave me. No matter what you are going through, always know that your life is valuable.

Things can change in a blink of an eye, but that does not mean you have to give up hope. I may have lost my entire left eye, but guess what? I can see life so much clearly now. You don't need a physical eye to see the goodness of God. Experiencing this new normal has allowed me to be closer to God. It has shown me that even when you go through difficult and challenging experiences, God is always there. He will never leave you nor forsake you and He can bring you through horrible circumstances. Through it all, He showed me that my life has purpose.

Through my pain He brought a message from my mess, a testimony from my test. Still, I rise!! I am like that Phoenix that rises from the ashes. And now, I'm soaring! Remember, it's not where you've been, it's where you are going. When you see me, you are looking at a miracle! I have had 13 reconstructive surgeries and 1 more coming soon. What strengthens me is knowing that through my story I can empower and motivate someone else to be a survivor and do what it takes to protect themselves from domestic violence.

Divannah Small is a wife, mother, sister, and friend living in Chicago, IL. She is a graduate of Harold Washington College with her Associates Degree in General Studies and Loyola University Chicago with her Bachelors in Management with plans to attend graduate school to pursue her MBA.

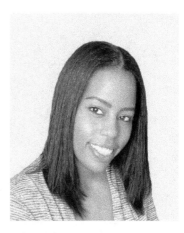

She has a heart for God and a passion to motivate and empower youth, particularly young women. She hopes to reach as many as she can through her personal testimony, writing, and motivational speaking. Her first book, From **Abandoned To Above**, focuses on helping youth rise above negative experiences in their lives and find purpose from their pain.

CHAPTER FIFTEEN

THE SET UP

BY DIVANNAH SMALL

If you only knew my story! They say to never judge a book by it's cover, and you really shouldn't! So, let me tell you about me. My cover looks pretty good from the outside. At first glance you would think I had it all together-- good looks, head on my shoulders, and seemingly happy-go-lucky. You would never know that as a baby I was diagnosed with fetal alcohol syndrome and a learning disability. You would never know that I had dyslexia and didn't learn how to read until the 1st grade via hooked on phonics. You would never know that I was physically and sexually abused as a child. You would never know it at first glance. We all have a Cover.

From the beginning, I was set up to fail in life. I experienced a lot of negativity as a child. In and out of foster homes, I always felt like I was a bad person and things were my fault. Rejection starts early. Actually, it can start in the womb and then our experience with it shapes our perception and outlook in life from childhood right into adulthood. It affects how we respond or don't respond to people. It jeopardizes our ability to cultivate healthy relationships. Rejection can cause us to not understand our true identity and purpose and lead to unhealthy connections and people-pleasing behaviors just to feel loved and accepted.

Going through what I did, I learned that what was meant for evil would ultimately be used for my good! I should have been another statistic, but God had other plans for me. *"For I know the thoughts that I think toward you, saith the Lord, thoughts of peace, and not of evil, to give you an expected end (Jeremiah 29:11 KJV)." Read that again!*

Okay, back to the story. Once I landed in my final foster home, my foster mother put me in school. I was deemed "special needs," but she would not settle for this diagnosis. She insisted that Chicago Public School (CPS) test my learning abilities differently. When they did, my journey in special needs did not last one hot second. Another failed setup.

After winning this battle, she then taught me how to read properly using *Hooked on Phonics*. Learning to read resulted in me rising to the top of my first-grade class! Talk about overcoming an obstacle! As I mentioned earlier, I also had been diagnosed with a writing disorder called Dyslexia. But somehow, I became ambidextrous. Another win! My learning disabilities were being overturned one by one going from having *special needs* to becoming an academic achiever!

By the time I reached the third grade, I had won my first spelling bee at school. Since then, I have continued to gather many more academic achievements. I am indeed a miracle through the grace of GOD! When it's all said and done, God has the FINAL say over our lives and what we will become! What we see or what others see is not what God sees! I am a testimony to this truth so I salute every person who has overcome *any* obstacle in their life. I encourage you to never give up on God or yourself. The setup is truly only a come up! So let me encourage you, *"Be strong and of a good courage, fear not, nor be afraid of them: for the Lord thy God, he it is that doth go with thee; he will not fail thee, nor forsake thee"* (See Joshua 1).

In Loving Memory of Lisa Boyd

A WOMAN OF FAITH

Our great desire is that you will keep on loving others as long as life lasts, in order to make certain that what you hope for will come true. Hebrews 11:6 NLT

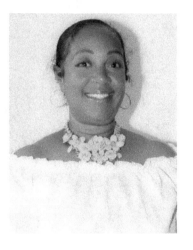

Lisa Boyd is inspired to live, enjoy, and fulfill the plan God has for her life. According to Jeremiah 29:11, God has a wonderful plan for all our lives. *Plans to prosper us and not to harm us; plans to give us hope for our future.*

In 2015, at 47 years old, Lisa was diagnosed with stage two triple negative Breast Cancer. As if fighting for her life wasn't enough, she lost her mother, her marriage, and her business while fighting Breast Cancer! The devil attacked her mentally, physically, and emotionally. But, she stood on her faith in God!

Knowing that God is a rewarder of all who diligently seek him (Hebrews 11:6), she remained steadfast and unmovable because she wanted to live and show forth God's glory to the world. According to John 11:14, *"All sickness is not unto death; but for the glory of God!"* We also know according to 1 Peter 5:10 that after a season of suffering, God in His grace will restore, confirm, strengthen, and establish you.

After surviving 6 months of chemotherapy, radiation and outpatient surgeries, Lisa received the healing in 2016 she was standing in faith for. Now she is not only a breast cancer survivor, she is an advocate for breast cancer awareness and offers support to others. She is the President and CEO of two small businesses, an author, a Certified Christian Counselor, and most importantly she's a humble servant of GOD.

Lisa jokingly agrees, *"That it was good that she was afflicted"* (Psalms 119:71). She believes the diagnosis was simply a test of her faith because she feared mammograms and therefore did not take them. After God rewarded her faithfulness, her faith and her relationship with Him enhanced tremendously! She humbly admits that she loves the woman she is becoming in Christ and she lives her life *inspired* by faith. www.BeInspiredByFaith.com

CHAPTER SIXTEEN

WALK BY FAITH

BY LISA BOYD

K eep your head up, your eyes forward and keep walking by faith. The Bible says that *"All things work together for the good of them that love the LORD and are called according to his purpose"* (Romans 8:28). In the words of Langston Hughes... "Life for me ain't been no crystal stair." I've had numerous encounters with fear where I had no other intelligent choice but to trust God and walk by faith (2 Corinthians 5:7).

My most fearful encounter was in 2015 when I was diagnosed with Breast Cancer. Everything I worked for and loved was falling apart right before my eyes. I was losing (almost) everything I valued. One day, I read something funny. It went like this, "If you want to make GOD laugh, tell Him your plans". That's not funny, that's actually very true. I'm a visionary. So, the majority of my adult life, I have been planning my life and my future the way I wanted it to be, without asking GOD anything! I had not practiced what God says in Matthew 6:33, *"Seek ye first and the kingdom of GOD, and his righteousness and all these things will be added to you."*

Proverbs 3:5 also instructs us to *"Trust in the LORD with all our heart; lean not to our OWN understanding, in all our ways ACKNOWLEDGE GOD and He will direct our path."* Not only did God leave us with His Word but He also gave us promises to stand on that require faith! I am so happy to be sharing this gospel (good news) with you. Although the devil afflicted my body with breast cancer, and sadly, I lost my business, my marriage, and my mother, my love for God and my faith in Him grew tremendously!

My mom's transition was the most heart-wrenching encounter (aside from my cancer diagnosis) I had experienced. I wrestled with anxiety attacks and severe depression. I had never had such encounters with grief ever before. But, I continued to trust God and walk by faith (Hebrews 11:6). At that point in my life, I drew closer to God and began asking Him for direction for my life. The Word of God tells us that *"If any man lacks WISDOM, ask for it"* (James 1:5).

In this season, I began asking God everything because I had no clue what I should do next. All I knew was that I wanted to live and not die, so I could share with unbelievers the benefits of having faith in God (Psalms 118:17). I discovered that God never allows pain without a purpose.

God also began to speak to me. He told me "To forgive." Forgive everyone that has hurt you. Keep your head up, look forward, get counseling, and stop dwelling on your past. With a little time, I learned to do exactly that. I had not realized how damaged my mental health was, but God knew. Doing the counseling sessions, I felt God repairing and realigning my life, mentally, physically, and emotionally because of my obedience to forgive. Since I've been healed, God is beautifully restoring my life. Faith in God changed my life. Whatever I can't change I don't worry about.

I currently have 2 small businesses that I love and enjoy. One is my inspirational T-shirt brand, "INSPIRED BY FAITH." It provides faith wear for the entire family. The other is my Breast Cancer Support Group and that is also "INSPIRED BY FAITH NFP." I faithfully visit the Cancer Treatment Center monthly to deliver chemo care packages to patients that are currently fighting breast cancer. I go to give them hope by sharing my testimony of faith with them. I want them to see that cancer doesn't mean the end of their lives.

I also partner with other NFP organizations that promote family & fairness in the world. Several weeks after beginning chemo, my sister and I organized a team of breast cancer supporters to walk annually in support of our mission and the Making Strides Against

Breast Cancer Foundation annual walks held during October in Chicago and Atlanta.

I have been the spokeswoman for several businesses supporting breast cancer awareness such as Violet Flower Shop summer community events (Berwyn, IL) and the Ashley Stewart Clothing Store for Breast Cancer Awareness Event held in October, (Atlanta GA). I have also been assigned speaking engagements, received honors and awards for my faith in the Lord, my courage in face of adversities, and my help in the community. I have been honored at the Dream Center Church of Atlanta and received the Women of Ages Queen's award in Chicago. I have shared my testimony and inspiration with Believers and Achievers Dental School, Full Gospel Church, Prayze Café Online Radio, Warrior Talk Online Radio,1690 WVON, IHeartRadio, and Making Headlines News Online news.

I faithfully attend and support my church, the Family Worship Center in Chicago, Illinois under the leadership of Bishop Noah Nicholson l, where I get an exceptional amount of good teaching and serve on several ministries including the Food Ministry (distributing food to the community), Hospitality, E-learning, Singles Ministry and wherever God has me to do. I now adjust my "scheduled" plans for God's will for my life because I know, God's plan is always what's BEST for me! Sometimes the plan and the process is painful and hard, but His plan for our lives is rewarding, fulfilling and better than we could have ever imagined (Ephesians 3:20)!

#GoneGirls be inspired and keep walking by faith!

Sharon D. Green is an author, creative writer, professor and speaker. She is the owner of SDG Freelance Writing Services and Lifter of my Head LLC, an organization and clothing brand dedicated to the holistic needs, inspiration, encouragement, and education for survivors of sexual 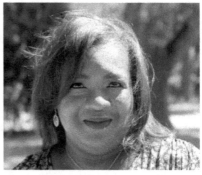 abuse/trauma, religious abuse/trauma, and depressive conditions. Sharon's passion is to educate, uplift, and assist with total life transformation by focusing on biblical and spiritual development, life skills, personal growth, and development. Her mission is to restore peoples' hope in God and the Bible despite what has happened to them in life.

Sharon holds a Bachelor's degree in English Literature from DePaul University and a Master's degree in Urban Leadership from Northern Baptist Theological Seminary. She is a member of New Life Covenant Church Southeast under the leadership of Pastor John F. Hannah where she is a trained Sunday school and discipleship teacher. Sharon resides in the Chicagoland area.

CHAPTER SEVENTEEN

THE ULTIMATE CRUTCH: MY VIEW OF GOD IN TIMES OF WEAKNESS

BY SHARON D. GREEN

As I reflect on an ankle injury I had a few years ago, I'm reminded of how much I needed and relied on my crutch. At first, the crutch was awkwardly helping my mobility. I didn't know how to use it properly in order to get the desired results I needed. One day a friend saw me struggling and walking awkwardly with my crutch. Without asking, he gently took my crutch, and showed me how to use it.

The fall and winter seasons of life bring greater opportunity for injuries. The coldness and iciness of life can lead to slips and falls, which cause injury. These are the seasons I have struggled the most with depressive conditions. However, my crutch has helped me to bear the weight of those seasons. The crutch, a mobility aid that transfers weight from the legs to the upper body, assists us when we're too weak or injured to walk.

I wondered why I held on to this crutch. Now I see that it reminds me of how I view God in seasons of weakness. There were times I didn't know how to take advantage of the Holy Spirit's presence and His help. Even in times of prayer, I struggled to believe and receive what Jesus had provided access for me to have. It took a skilled leader to show me how to view God correctly, and how to walk with Him through the daily moments of life. Just like I relied on my crutch then, I rely on God now. I hold on to Him for mobility. Holding onto God gives me security and stability, so I don't fall down and injure myself. When I'm tired and weak, I lean further into Him for more strength and support. I allow Him to bear the weight of life while He's holding me up.

Sometimes, I look over to Him just to make sure He's still there, just in case I need more of Him. I look over to Him to remind me of what He's already done for me, how He keeps me sound and steady as I walk with Him. This is one of the many ways I stay delivered of depressive conditions. I encourage you to rely on and lean into God today.

Give God your whole heart, no matter how damaged it may be to you. To God, you're already perfect! Allow God to guard your heart for you, and trust that He won't fail you. Submit your entire life to Him, no matter fragile. Little by little, you will notice joy and strength as you walk with Him through life. God is good and He loves you unconditionally. Believe me, you can trust Him!

Desiree McCray, also known as Minister Des, is a young prophetic voice for this generation. Along with preaching and ministering, Des is a poet, painter, published author, and host of the podcast titled "PROPHETIC SISTA GIRL." She graduated in 2018 from the University of Missouri in Columbia, Missouri with a Bachelor of Arts in English—Creative Writing. An 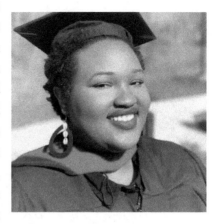 award-winning preacher, Minister Des is a 2021 graduate with a Master of Divinity from Princeton Theological Seminary in Princeton, New Jersey. Des McCray seeks to make the gospel real and relevant by providing spiritual affirmation, divine inspiration, and radical transformation through the word of God.

CHAPTER EIGHTEEN

MEDITATION:
A CREDIBLE WITNESS
BY DESIREE MCCRAY

16 For we did not follow cleverly devised stories when we told you about the coming of our Lord Jesus Christ in power, but we were eyewitnesses of his majesty. 17 He received honor and glory from God the Father when the voice came to him from the Majestic Glory, saying, "This is my Son, whom I love; with him I am well pleased."[a] 18 We ourselves heard this voice that came from heaven when we were with him on the sacred mountain.

19 We also have the prophetic message as something completely reliable, and you will do well to pay attention to it, as to a light shining in a dark place, until the day dawns and the morning star rises in your hearts. 20 Above all, you must understand that no prophecy of Scripture came about by the prophet's own interpretation of things. 21 For prophecy never had its origin in the human will, but prophets, though human, spoke from God as they were carried along by the Holy Spirit.

2 Peter 1:16-21 NIV

If you have ever watched a murder mystery or action film, then you know that a hit-man's job is to kill witnesses because the witness is a key element in developing the story. Eyewitnesses can produce very compelling testimony. Eyewitness testimony is critically important to the justice system, but also in the kingdom of God. Likewise, your witness is a powerful part of developing the story of God's glory.

When I was about 10 years old, I was bullied for my hair, my clothes, and my size. I've always been a plus-size person. Even in my little body, I was full of God, preaching mini-sermons in aftercare at school. I realized the bullies and cruel kids were trying to steal and kill my witness because it was potent to encourage other people.

Somewhere in the world is someone who needs to hear your testimony. You have experienced God truly, not as a result of "cleverly devised stories" (2 Peter 1:16). No one can tell your story like you can. Peter allowed Jesus's death to kill his witness and he denied Christ three times. Forbid anything or anyone from being a hitman to your eyewitness. Many people will come to know God better through your sharing some of what God has done, even if there are not enough hours in the day to tell it all.

Be an eyewitness to the Lord's majesty. Reject the shame and guilt of your past, as Peter did. Peter ultimately became the rock of Christ's church. Do not let your history silence your destiny. Be strengthened by the reminder of your power as a living testimony to God's transformative grace.

Shalonda Blackwell was born and raised on the west side of Chicago. She attended Genevieve Melody School where she was valedictorian of her 8th grade class. She went on to study at Charles P. Steinmetz High School. By the time she was 16 years old, she became pregnant. She dropped out of high school at the age of 17.

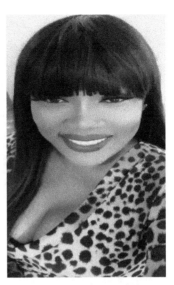

Determined to get her high school education, Shalonda managed to immediately pass the GED exam. At the age of 22, she attended Robert Morris College where she obtained her Bachelor's degree in Business Management. Later, she attended Keller Graduate School of Management where she earned her Masters degree in Business and Masters in Human Resource Management proving she is a firm believer in hard work and overcoming obstacles.

As a youth, she attended The Amazing Church of God in Christ where the Elder Jefferson Campbell presided. Throughout her teen years and beyond, she attended Truth and Deliverance International Ministries where Apostle John T. Abercrombie, Jr. is pastor. Although shy, Shalonda loves to sing. As a soloist, she has led praise and worship and sung in the choir for many years.

Shalonda is also a philanthropist. As a teenage mother, she experienced hardships, so she believes in helping others and mentoring younger women. Shalonda has a giving heart and you can see her generosity at work in her gifts to homeless shelters and the baskets she builds which contain hygiene products and other essentials for those in need.

CHAPTER NINETEEN

OUT OF ORDER

BY SHALONDA BLACKWELL

W hen I think about it, I've never done anything in my life in the typical order society, or my family for that matter, felt that I should. I had a child at 16, got married at 19, and went to college at 22. I was able to successfully complete my goals, just not in the chronological order expected of me.

By the time I was 25, I married again. By then, I had 2 children and none were by my current husband. I remember when my husband and I met. His mother wasn't very fond of me. She had a way of letting me know that she didn't approve of me being with her son. I was a young woman with 2 children trying to find my way, albeit still out of order. I was reminded of the scripture in Psalm 37:23, *"The steps of a good man are ordered by the Lord: and he delighteth in his way."*

When my second husband and I had been married for about 2 years, we welcomed his only son. I discovered this too wasn't something his mother would approve of. She jokingly made comments about my son's eyes and how he didn't look like his father. Over the years, I developed ill-feelings towards her due to all her negative comments and antics. I wanted her to stop with the foolishness and accept me as her daughter-in-law just as my family had accepted her son as their own. I tried everything I knew how to get her to like me, but nothing worked. She would be nice for a short period of time, only to revert to her previous behaviors.

After about 18 years of marriage, I had learned that I had developed an aggressive form of breast cancer. The kind where statistics proved that only 25% of those diagnosed, survive. Because I had grown up in the church, I knew that God could heal me. I kept the faith, kept it moving, and God did just that! As I write this, I am going into my 3rd year cancer free! During all this time his mother has never reached out, never asked how I was doing. I almost felt like there might have been a smug grin on her face when she learned that I had been diagnosed. I never told my husband, but it was something that I had noticed.

A few months ago, in April of 2021 to be exact, my husband found his mother in a desperate situation where she needed to be hospitalized immediately. He made sure she got the best care possible. She had gone into the hospital a few times in the past for various ailments, so we did not think her condition was something to be gravely concerned about. But after various tests and multiple doctor's visits, we learned that his mother had an aggressive form of cancer which was affecting her lungs, kidney, and liver. The doctors informed us that she had only months to live and that she would need to be on hospice care.

As you can imagine, we were both shocked. This was so unexpected. My husband immediately looked to me to assist in getting things started. His mother had made the demands that she wanted to be home and not at a facility. We brought her to our home. Even while she was in hospice and in a dying state, she was still mean, nasty and disapproving of me as his wife. There I was a woman who loved her husband in a situation with someone who hated me. Did my husband really expect me to change her diapers, feed, and tend to her while he worked?

I thought to myself about all the things that she had done and said to me over the years. The mistreatment that I didn't deserve all because I didn't measure up to her expectations of whom she wanted her son to marry. She was now in my home and I had to take care of her. I looked to the heavens and said, "God, you really got good jokes!" When I think about how good God has been to me in my own life, I couldn't dare to do to her what she had done to me. Galatians 6:7 came to mind, *"Be not deceived; God is not mocked: for whatsoever a man soweth, that shall he also reap."*

Based on the order of God, I took care of her. I made sure that the doctors, nurses, and staff did what they were supposed to. On numerous occasions, I went in and watched movies, fed, sang, and praised God with her while she stayed with us. On her last day, I went into her room and held her hand. It was as if she knew that she was transitioning. She held my hand so tightly that day but didn't speak. She passed away on July 4, 2021. I knew that she was with God. To be absent from the body is to be present with the Lord! I was glad that I had a chance to serve God and learn true humility.

Doris J Williams is a licensed Evangelist, Elder, and Prophetess. She is a motivation to the body of Christ and a prophetic voice. Doris loves what she does as an encourager and a spiritual midwife even when obstacles are presented before her. One thing for sure, Doris will still encourage you to press forward and help to push you in the direction of deliverance. Doris does not take any part of her calling lightly. In ministry for over 26 years, she has experienced many challenges, but she has stayed the course and continues to press on. Doris writes expressively and prophetically and this is just an excerpt of one assignment of many books that will be released. Look for more from her ministry on Facebook page, Sista's Empowerment Circle, Prayer Healing and Deliverance Prophetess Doris J. Williams. As a person with many gifts, she is an entrepreneur, creative, and Etiquette Director. Most importantly, she is an overcomer and an example of what God can do.

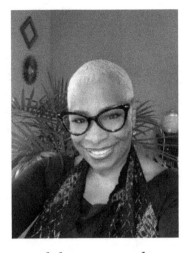

Prophétesses Doris J Williams
Email djww52@gmail.com
Instagram Ms_Defined
Facebook Prophetess DJ Williams Ministries

CHAPTER TWENTY

FROM BROKEN TO BETTER

BY PROPHETESS DORIS J WILLIAMS

And the vessel that he made of clay was marred in the hand of
the potter: so he made it again another vessel, as seemed good to
the potter to make it. Jeremiah 18:4

As you read, I want to encourage you that a healing will take place within you and God will release a refreshing in your spirit as He did for me. I didn't know when I was going to get to the place where I stopped bleeding. But God did it! I'm healed and whole to release the gift God has given me for this world. I was once in a broken place that gripped me with hurt so badly that I just wanted to shut people out of my life, church folk in particular. I have to tell the truth to stay free.

I wanted to do God's work, but only for people I selected. Well, that's not how it works when you are called to the nation. The enemy knows what your purpose is, but he does not know God's plan. That's why the Word of God says in Jeremiah 29:11, *"I know the plans I have for you."* God knows the outcome already, we just have to stick to what He says and do it. Will it be easy? I don't believe it's easy, but what I can say is that it strengthens you for your process to fulfill the purpose according to His plan.

I was broken from marriage manipulation and relationship abuse (mentally, spiritually, and sometimes, even physically). I almost became confused from what I knew to do and what I was allowing to push me on the edge. I'm going to say this right here, whatever you go through, stay spiritual. I was talked down to, talked at, and held back from progressing in areas of my life only because I allowed it. So, I blame nobody for what I had the power over.

But when you relinquish yourself to people, you give up a part of you that is vulnerable and open to be used. This lesson of brokenness reminds me whose I am and who I am. I take every scripture to heart like it's a screenshot that I have to keep pasting daily in my affairs. Now I learn to guard my heart as I put my trust only in the Lord. This has made me better for my purpose and more mature in my walk. However, when the enemy came to shake me and traumatize me in a way that I could never imagine, I could hear the Lord saying "Hold on, this is to shake you and cause a break. I'm the one that will allow your break for the better you to come forth. You know sometimes you have to break open the oyster shell to see the pearl."

We are jewels and every jewel has to be carved out of stone or come out of something precious. I realized my traumatization was attributed to me actually being broken and I needed to be healed. Even in my broken state I knew I had God's grace upon my life. As an intercessor called to prayer, an Evangelist called to preaching, and a Prophetess with utterance the Lord allows me to release, I knew then that my trauma was designed for me to give up on God. Sometimes when we are faced with trauma it causes us to lose sight of the very one who has the ability to guide us through the situation.

Again, I'm going to say, let this message ring out in your ears and take root in your spirit. Stay spiritual and do not be carnal-minded in your daily walk. The flesh gets easily offended and wants to react to the attack, but the Spirit of God in you will guide you through your hurt to your healing place. No weapon formed against you shall be able to prosper. As a matter of fact, keep looking towards God. When you are pressed in such a way that you feel trapped with no way out, remember that "Many are the afflictions of the righteous but the Lord will deliver you out of them all" (Psalms 34:18).

Lean in on God, cry out, and spare not. I cried many times asking God, why? In the same breath, I told God thank you as He kept revealing why. I want to encourage you that whatever you're going through, God will see you through to release your testimony as an overcomer. Your breaking is for the better in your making. You are a Queen. You are of a royal priesthood and a designer original. God has created you on purpose for His purpose and according to His plan.

I'm saying I used to feel broken, hurt, abandoned, and rejected. I felt misused and abused after I had given so much time to the marriage, ministry, and people. I had put too much trust in everything and everyone else and I believe this was God telling me to turn back to him, and seek His face. The funny thing is when you think that a situation is breaking you, it's really God breaking you in the situation for your breakthrough. God was preparing me all the time. When He was breaking me, He was also making me into the better woman I am right now. Everything that happened to me God had already shown me, so I was not shocked. I just shifted into my purpose.

When something happened that was supposed to be devastating, God's grace covered me. I had a divine breakthrough. I found myself again. I was able to see who I really was in God. I didn't realize that I was so lost and broken until I had to really seek God to find where He was taking me. What I found out about God is that He won't show you where He's taking you until He shows you who you are. That is so you can know why the purpose inside of you is being fulfilled in the designated place where He is calling you. The Lord really had to work on me in my brokenness. I was so messed up that I didn't want to hear the church name mentioned or anybody that was associated with the church. I didn't want to see them and I didn't want them to see me. And then one day I told God, "Hide me from my enemies and heal me."

At that point, I realized after years of bondage in a marriage of manipulation, my wound was deeper than what was on the surface. I know when God calls you, He covers you even when you don't think you're worthy. He said I will put you underneath my wings and that's what He did for me through this process of brokenness. I just wanted to get better and after eight years of unforgiveness in my heart. That was when God revealed that my pain was for the purpose of the healing of other women and I had to forgive to heal. The process would not be easy, but He would bring me through to make me better.

I fasted, prayed, and cried out again to God telling him this time I wanted to trust and forgive. I didn't like the way I felt knowing that I was called to the nation to preach, pray, and prophesy. I became fully aware that the enemy was out to kill, steal, and destroy what God had placed inside of me.

God kept me through it all when it looked like I should've lost my mind. God was regulating my mind. Where my heart seemed like it was broken, God was really fixing my heart. Where my spirit looked like it should've been messed up, God was renewing my spirit. So, I went from broken to better! God provided for me. He placed my feet on the rock and made me better so I could tell my story to encourage and empower women.

Today I am fulfilling my purpose. I am the founder of Sista's Empowerment Circle on Facebook and I serve in the ministry of Prayer Healing and Deliverance with Prophetess Doris Williams. This is who God has called me to be in this hour and I just want to encourage you today to trust in the Lord with your whole heart and lean not to your own understanding, but acknowledge him in everything that you do he will direct your paths. You will come out on top. That is your best choice because giving up is never an option when God is leading and directing you.

Don't let a day go by without asking God what he requires of you. Don't live your life according to man's expectation, but according to what God requires of you. I learned how to trust in Jesus and how to trust in God. He showed me how to guard my heart and to be effective in my prayers knowing that when I call upon his name He will respond.

CHAPTER TWENTY-ONE

IT ALMOST TOOK ME OUT

BY VERONDA MCKENNIE-WILLIAMS

Life has a way of throwing bricks right at you. However, it needs to happen. I needed to find out who I was, how much strength I had and exactly how necessary my relationship with God is and means to my life. I have a calling on my life, just like you have a calling on your life. Each of us have been given gifts at conception. We read in Jeremiah 1:5, *"Before I formed thee in the belly I knew thee; and before thou camest forth out of the womb I sanctified thee, and I ordained thee a prophet unto the nations."*

GOD knows who you are and what His desire is for our lives. In fact, He has good plans for us. Jeremiah 29:11 tells us, *"For I know the thoughts (plans) that I think toward you, saith the Lord, thoughts of peace, and not of evil, to give you an expected end.* But if you are distracted and overwhelmed, you will miss it.

I was always praying over others and their calling, but I forgot about me. I was always helping others and coming to their rescue without taking time for myself. I was drowning. I was losing my breath and sinking to the bottom fast with no one to help me. This drained me physically, mentally, and emotionally. Something had to be different. "GOD save me" was my prayer, my cry, my plea. "Help me!" My life depended on it.

Life has a way of knocking you right off your square. I wanted the perfect life, family, and friends. I almost had it. Then life hit me with the resurfacing of childhood trauma and bad decisions. Those bad decisions came with a price as we read in the book of Romans," For *the wages of sin is death; but the gift of God is eternal life through Jesus Christ our Lord" (Romans 6:23).*

I struggled with loss of self-esteem and then divorce, which at that time of my life was the ultimate traumatic experience. It almost took me out. Death hit my home. Not physical death, but because of my decisions, a death of my finances, lifestyle, relationships, and marriage. Sometimes you can try to live a life that was never meant for you. You weren't meant to live a life of poverty, a life in the streets, or a life exposed to drugs and alcoholism. You open the door for sin and distractions. As best said in 1 John 2:16, *"For all that is in the world, the lust of the flesh, and the lust of the eyes, and the pride of life, is not of the Father but is of the world."* These are all distractions from the life you are supposed to live.

I have been a hoarder and procrastinator. This means more than holding on to material possessions and moving slowly. I was holding on to pain, lies, rejection, abandonment, disappointment, deception, thoughts of suicide, and mental and physical abuse. I was mentally exhausted. My life had to be drastically disrupted. I got knocked down and broken down.

I was broken. I walked right into solitude and depression and then shut everyone out. I needed a transfusion. Cleanse me, O God! I walked into my wilderness and my own "Job experience," remembering that he lost everything he had, except his faith in God. But also remember, Job gained double for his trouble. That brings to mind the verse in *Isaiah 54:17: "No weapon that is formed against thee shall prosper; and every tongue that shall rise against thee in judgment thou shalt condemn. This is the heritage of the servants of the Lord, and their righteousness is of me, saith the Lord."*

No matter who turned against Job, no matter what Job initially lost, GOD restored him and all that he had lost. You've got to hold on to the Word of God through your wilderness and your "Job experience." I had to hold on to what I was taught. This is why I went to church and Sunday school for all those years. It wasn't just to socialize, participate in programs, sing in the choir, or attend events.

Here is the test: would you still love yourself, when others don't see you in a positive light? When others walk away from you? If you lost all your worldly riches and possessions? How will you deal with your shame and your bad decisions? Well, your test will let you know. It will expose any weakness or strengths you have.

All of this was God's way of emptying me out. My life was redirected and refocused. But we sometimes miss it because we don't want to come face to face with the situation and be honest about what's happening. You have to be honest. If you miss it, you have to repeat the test. During my test I prayed more. I built a healthy coping mechanism to keep my mind from being idle. This process built me. I had to go back and fix my broken places. It made me an overcomer. It taught me things about myself, others connected to me, and those who should be connected to me. I was always optimistic and positive and a tad bit naïve. I didn't want to accept the truth about others and definitely didn't want to accept the truth about me and this stage in life.

When you don't value yourself, anybody or anything can distract you. Know your worth. Don't let any abuse mentally, physically, emotionally, or spiritually make you forget your worth. You are worth it. You are worth being loved, celebrated, and honored. You don't have to settle for anything less. You can have love, success, happiness and real joy.

During those times I didn't realize my own calling outside of wife, mother, sister, daughter, friend or whatever capacity others needed me. Then I came to myself. God awakened me to realize the calling on my life. I had to focus on myself and do a self-evaluation. I realized I was worthy of living, being happy, and becoming all that I desired to be. I needed to walk in my calling because I was worth it all, despite my trials and tribulations. Despite the circumstances, I deserved to live and have life more abundantly as Jesus promised in *John 10:10*, "*The thief (circumstances) cometh not, but for to steal, and to kill, and to destroy: I am come that they might have life, and that they might have it more abundantly.*"

Always remember, you deserve more. You deserve to live, and you deserve to start again! Get up and start again. I know it will work for your good because God's Word promises it will. *"And we know that all things work together for good to them that love God, to them who are the called according to his purpose"* (Romans 8:28).

Then you will be able to share your testimony of how you've overcome. Remember we overcome by the word of our testimony. Therefore, be careful what you say. Words have power. If you want God to move on your behalf, only speak the Word of God and walk in your authority. You are resilient. You have endurance. You are an overcomer. You are the lender and not the borrower. You are the head and not the tail. Watch God do just what he promised. Stand on the promises of God!

God reminded me that we are resilient, we can endure and we can overcome. Say it with me: I am resilient, I can endure, I will overcome. Stand on the promises of GOD. Be the Noah of your time. People will only believe you when you build it and the rain comes. Build your life. Build your dream. What do you believe about you? What do you believe GOD said about you? You work it and GOD will bless it!

Delores Erin Hood was born out of a loving marital union. Isaac and Corrine Hood were more than delighted to finally have their daughter after bringing five wonderful sons into the world. With her mother being an educator, Delores excelled in school academically. She graduated from Westinghouse Vocational High School on Chicago's west side with high marks. Adult life came upon her fast and Delores chose the fast route. But the God that sits high and looks low always took special care of her, 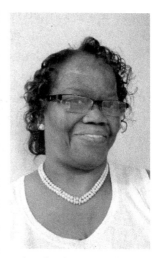 knowing that one day she would use her spiritual gifts for His glory!

Delores began her work for the Master at The Salvation Army Temple Corps in 1988. There she dedicated her life to the troubled youth in the community through several programs designed to help young ladies become successful women. She also worked with senior citizens who would have otherwise had no one to assist them with grocery shopping, doctors' visits, etc. Delores was a member of The Salvation Army Madison Street Choir, one of the first choirs to be formed within the Salvation Army's Chicago area.

When Delores came into contact with Victorious Christian Fellowship (VCF) under the leadership and direction of Bishop Victor W. and Apostle Vivian L. Harris, she knew it was time to move on, but she left a piece of her heart with the Temple Corps. Although she had already been introduced to God's word, she really got to know Him through the extensive and eye-opening lessons she has received and still receives through the worship, preaching, and teaching at VCF *where victory is learned . . .not by chance!* At VCF Delores helped around the church and was available to do whatever was needed to give Bishop and Apostle Harris personal assistance. After they passed away, Delores began serving with Pastor Robert and Pastor Angela Johnson at Greater Love Great Works Outreach International.

Delores is gifted to work with those that are living with physical disadvantages. She currently works at Oak Trace Health Center, helping the residents with bathing, medication, and basic living needs. She knows in her heart that her calling is serving and helping others and she does it with great joy. God has blessed Delores beyond words in the present and she wholeheartedly awaits what's to come in the future.

Continuing in His service!

CHAPTER TWENTY-TWO

SO MANY TIMES I CRIED

BY DELORES ERIN HOOD

God works in mysterious ways. Being hurt by the leadership in a church really took its toll on me. It made my heart heavy. Many nights I cried out to God. My experience with the church leadership exposed unfairness, jealousy, envy, selfishness, and degradation.

Despite everything I went through, I became stronger. To God be the glory!

I stayed in the storm and cried out to God many times, knowing I wanted to leave the church. Unbeknownst to me, God had a plan. It took obedience for me to realize that God will allow us to be in an uncomfortable place to elevate us to the next level. No matter what circumstance we find ourselves in, we can take comfort in this promise from Isaiah 41:10,*"Fear thou not, for I am with thee: be not dismayed; for I am thy God. I will strengthen thee: yea, I will help thee; yea, I will uphold thee with the right hand of my righteousness."*

You must always recognize who you're working with, and understand who you're working for.....God! By my faith, God helped me through the storm. No matter what problems arise, He is there to help us overcome the torment, scars, and hurt. With my faith and God's help, I am able to encourage others today.

Continue the journey to complete this devotional. Write your story give it to Jesus, He cares and He is a Healer.

_____

_____

_____

_____

_____

_____

_____

_____

_____

_____

_____

_____

_____

_____

_____

_____

_____

_____

_____

_____

_____

_____

_____

_____

_____

_____

_____

In Loving Memory

of

DeLanda M. Llyod-Hamilton

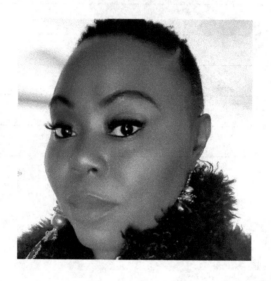

#GONE GIRL NOTES

#GONE GIRL NOTES

#GONE GIRL NOTES

#GONE GIRL NOTES

#GONE GIRL NOTES

#GONE GIRL NOTES